Morgellons Disease

The Importance of Early Treatment for Morgellons Disease

By

Eoin Fintan
Copyright@2023

Table of Contents

CHAPTER 1
Introduction

1.1 What is Morgellons

Morgellons, also known as Morgellons disease, is a perplexing and controversial medical condition characterized by a range of unusual and often distressing symptoms. The hallmark of Morgellons is the presence of fibers or filaments that protrude from the skin. These fibers are typically colored white, black, blue, or red and are often accompanied by sensations of itching, crawling, and stinging. Affected individuals may describe these fibers as emerging from or embedded in their skin, and they may believe that these fibers are connected to their symptoms.

In addition to the fibers, Morgellons is associated with a myriad of other symptoms, which can vary greatly from person to person. These symptoms can include skin lesions, rashes, joint pain, fatigue, cognitive difficulties, and psychiatric manifestations such as anxiety and depression. Some individuals with Morgellons also report the presence of tiny, colored granules or specks in their skin.

Morgellons is a poorly understood condition, and its etiology remains a subject of debate and research. The medical community has struggled to provide a definitive explanation for the disease, which has led to skepticism and controversy. Many individuals with Morgellons have reported difficulty obtaining a clear diagnosis and appropriate treatment from healthcare professionals. The lack of a widely accepted medical framework for Morgellons has made it challenging for patients to receive the support and care they need.

1.2 Importance of Early Treatment

The importance of early treatment for Morgellons cannot be overstated, even in the face of the controversy surrounding the condition. While medical understanding of Morgellons is limited, and the cause remains uncertain, it is evident that individuals who experience Morgellons symptoms often face a significant reduction in their quality of life. Early intervention can have several crucial benefits:

1. **Symptom Management**: Morgellons symptoms, including skin discomfort, itching, and psychological distress, can be extremely debilitating. Early treatment can help manage these symptoms, alleviating the suffering experienced by affected individuals.

2. **Prevention of Complications**: Left untreated, Morgellons symptoms can lead to complications such as skin infections from excessive scratching and open sores. Addressing these issues early can prevent these secondary health problems.

3. **Psychological Support**:
Morgellons can have a
profound impact on an
individual's mental health.
Early treatment can provide
psychological support,
including counseling and
therapies, to help patients cope
with the emotional toll of their
condition.

4. **Patient Advocacy**: Early
diagnosis and treatment can
empower individuals with
Morgellons to become
advocates for their own health.
It can also help raise awareness
within the medical community,
potentially leading to improved
research and understanding of
the condition.

5. **Improved Quality of Life**:
While Morgellons may not yet

have a definitive cure, early treatment can help individuals regain some semblance of normalcy in their lives. Managing symptoms and receiving support can lead to an improved quality of life.

It is important to acknowledge that the controversy surrounding Morgellons has created challenges for both patients and healthcare providers. Some healthcare professionals may be hesitant to diagnose and treat the condition due to the lack of a clear medical consensus. However, early intervention, even if it involves symptom management and psychological support, can make a significant difference for individuals living with Morgellons. It is crucial to approach this condition with empathy, understanding, and a commitment to alleviating the suffering of those affected.

CHAPTER 2

Understanding Morgellons

2.1 Morgellons Symptoms

Morgellons is characterized by a wide range of symptoms that can vary from person to person, making it a challenging condition to define. While the presence of fibers or filaments in or on the skin is a hallmark feature, individuals with Morgellons often experience a constellation of other symptoms, including:

- **Skin Lesions and Rashes:** Morgellons patients frequently report the development of skin lesions and rashes. These may appear as open sores, red or inflamed areas, or ulcerations. The lesions are often accompanied by itching and discomfort.

- **Fiber-Like Structures:** The fibers associated with Morgellons can be colored white, black, blue, or red. They are often perceived as emerging from or embedded in the skin. These fibers are a primary source of concern for those with Morgellons.

- **Sensations of Crawling and Itching:** Affected individuals commonly describe sensations of something crawling on or under their skin. This crawling or itching sensation can be maddening and is a source of considerable distress.

- **Joint Pain and Fatigue:** Many Morgellons patients report joint pain and chronic fatigue. These symptoms can significantly impact a person's mobility and daily functioning.

- **Cognitive and Psychiatric Symptoms:** Cognitive difficulties, such as brain fog, memory problems, and difficulties concentrating, are often reported. Additionally, some patients experience psychiatric symptoms like anxiety, depression, and mood disturbances.

- **Presence of Colored Granules:** Some individuals report the presence of tiny colored granules or specks on or in their skin. These granules are often associated with the perception of a parasitic infection.

It's important to note that these symptoms are highly distressing to those experiencing them. They can have a profound impact on a person's quality of life, contributing to significant emotional and psychological distress.

2.2 Causes and Controversies

The exact causes of Morgellons remain a subject of debate and controversy within the medical community. Several theories have been proposed, including:

- **Delusional Parasitosis:** Some healthcare professionals and researchers have suggested that Morgellons may be a form of delusional parasitosis, a psychiatric condition in which individuals believe they are infested with parasites despite lacking evidence. However, this explanation does not account for the physical presence of fibers and other physical symptoms often observed in Morgellons patients.

- **Environmental Factors:** Some researchers have explored the possibility of environmental factors, such as exposure to toxins or infectious agents, contributing to Morgellons. Environmental triggers could play a role in the development of symptoms.

- **Psychological and Stress-Related Factors:** Stress and psychological distress are common among Morgellons patients. It's possible that these factors contribute to symptom exacerbation or that they are a consequence of living with a chronic and poorly understood condition.

Despite these theories, the precise etiology of Morgellons remains unclear, and no single cause has been definitively identified. This lack of consensus has contributed to the ongoing controversy surrounding the condition.

2.3 Diagnosis and Misdiagnosis

Diagnosing Morgellons is challenging due to the diverse and often subjective nature of the symptoms. Medical professionals typically use a process of exclusion to rule out other potential causes for the symptoms, such as dermatological conditions, infectious diseases, or underlying psychiatric disorders.

Misdiagnosis is not uncommon in cases of Morgellons, with some individuals being mistakenly labeled as having delusional parasitosis or other psychiatric conditions. This can lead to frustration and further stigmatization for patients.

Accurate diagnosis and appropriate care are essential to addressing Morgellons effectively. Healthcare providers need to approach the condition with an open mind, empathetic communication, and a willingness to collaborate with patients to manage their symptoms and improve their quality of life. It's also crucial for ongoing research to shed light on the underlying causes of Morgellons and develop evidence-based treatments.

CHAPTER 3

Conventional Medical Approaches

3.1 Medications and Topical Treatments

Conventional medical approaches to managing Morgellons often focus on addressing specific symptoms and providing relief to patients. Medications and topical treatments are commonly employed in this regard:

- **Antipruritic Medications:** Itching and discomfort are prevalent in Morgellons, and antipruritic medications such as antihistamines or corticosteroid creams may be prescribed to alleviate these symptoms.

- **Pain Management:** For individuals experiencing joint pain and discomfort, pain-relief medications may be recommended. Non-steroidal anti-inflammatory drugs (NSAIDs) are often considered.

- **Topical Skin Treatments:** Topical treatments, such as emollients and moisturizers, may be suggested to soothe and hydrate the skin, which can help with the healing of lesions.

- **Antibiotics:** In some cases, antibiotics may be prescribed to address any secondary skin infections that can arise from open sores or lesions due to excessive scratching.

Antibiotics are not a direct treatment for Morgellons itself but can be necessary to prevent complications.

It's important to note that these medications and treatments primarily aim to manage the symptoms of Morgellons rather than addressing the root cause of the condition, as the underlying cause remains uncertain.

3.2 Dermatological Procedures

Dermatological procedures may be considered in cases of Morgellons to address skin lesions and improve skin health. These procedures are typically performed by dermatologists and may include:

- **Debridement:** Removal of damaged or infected skin tissue, often necessary for managing open sores and lesions.

- **Biopsies:** A biopsy involves the removal of a small sample of skin tissue for examination under a microscope. While this may not provide a specific diagnosis of Morgellons, it can help rule out other skin conditions.

- **Wound Care:** Dermatologists can provide specialized wound care, which may include wound dressings, sutures, or other interventions to promote the healing of skin lesions.

Dermatological procedures are part of the broader effort to manage the physical aspects of Morgellons and prevent complications associated with skin issues.

3.3 Psychological Support

Psychological support is a crucial component of the conventional medical approach to Morgellons, given the emotional and psychological distress often experienced by patients. This support can take various forms:

- **Counseling and Therapy:** Mental health professionals, such as psychologists or psychiatrists, can provide counseling and therapy to help patients cope with the psychological challenges of living with Morgellons. Cognitive-behavioral therapy (CBT) is one approach that may be beneficial in addressing anxiety and depression.

- **Support Groups:** Morgellons support groups can be valuable for patients, as they offer a sense of community and a safe space to share experiences, feelings, and coping strategies.

- **Education and Empowerment:** Informing patients about the condition and its complexities can be empowering. Understanding that they are not alone and that there are healthcare professionals who are willing to help can significantly improve the psychological well-being of those with Morgellons.

Psychological support plays a vital role in improving the overall quality of life for individuals with Morgellons, as it can help manage the distress and anxiety that often accompanies this poorly understood condition.

CHAPTER 4

Alternative and Complementary Therapies

4.1 Diet and Nutrition

Diet and nutrition play a significant role in the management of Morgellons. While there are no specific dietary guidelines or treatments proven to cure Morgellons, some individuals with the condition have reported benefits from dietary changes. Here are some considerations:

- **Anti-Inflammatory Diet:** An anti-inflammatory diet, which focuses on foods that reduce inflammation in the body, may be helpful. This includes foods rich in omega-3 fatty acids, such as fatty fish (salmon, mackerel), as well as plenty of fruits and vegetables.

- **Hydration:** Staying well-hydrated is essential for overall health and can contribute to healthier skin. Drinking an adequate amount of water each day is recommended.

- **Avoiding Trigger Foods:** Some individuals with Morgellons report that certain foods or food additives can exacerbate their symptoms. Keeping a food diary and identifying potential trigger foods can be beneficial.

- **Supplements:** Some individuals may choose to take dietary supplements, such as vitamins and minerals, to support their overall health. It's important to consult with a healthcare professional before starting any supplementation regimen.

It's essential to approach dietary changes with caution and consult a healthcare provider or a registered dietitian for personalized advice. Additionally, keep in mind that dietary interventions are often used in conjunction with other treatment strategies and should not be considered a standalone solution for Morgellons.

4.2 Detoxification Strategies

Detoxification strategies are sometimes explored by individuals with Morgellons as a way to rid the body of potential toxins or pathogens that are believed to be associated with the condition. It's important to note that the efficacy and safety of detoxification methods are subject to debate and vary widely. Some detoxification strategies include:

- **Chelation Therapy:** Chelation therapy involves the use of substances that bind to heavy metals in the body and facilitate their elimination. This is often used in cases where heavy metal toxicity is suspected, but it should only be done under the guidance of a healthcare professional.

- **Colon Cleanses:** Some people consider colon cleansing or colon hydrotherapy to remove toxins from the digestive tract. These procedures are not supported by mainstream medical organizations and can have risks.

- **Sauna Therapy:** Sweating in a sauna is believed by some to help remove toxins from the body. It's important to use saunas safely and stay well-hydrated during and after sauna sessions.

- **Fasting:** Fasting or restricted diets may be attempted as a detoxification strategy. These approaches should be done under medical supervision and may not be suitable for everyone, especially those with medical conditions.

Detoxification strategies should be approached with caution, as they can carry potential risks and may not provide substantial benefits for individuals with Morgellons. It is advisable to consult with a healthcare provider before pursuing any detoxification regimen to ensure that it is safe and appropriate for your specific circumstances. Additionally, patients are encouraged to seek evidence-based treatments and consult with healthcare professionals who are knowledgeable about Morgellons.

4.3 Herbal and Natural Remedies

Herbal and natural remedies are often considered by individuals with Morgellons as alternative treatment options. While the efficacy of these remedies is not well-established, some people report finding relief from certain symptoms through the use of herbal and natural products. Here are some examples:

- **Topical Herbal Applications:** Some individuals apply herbal creams or ointments containing ingredients like aloe vera, calendula, or chamomile to soothe irritated skin and alleviate itching.

- **Herbal Supplements:** Herbal supplements, such as garlic, oregano oil, and turmeric, are believed by some to have antibacterial and anti-inflammatory properties and may be used to support overall health.

- **Essential Oils:** Essential oils like tea tree oil and lavender oil are occasionally used topically for their perceived calming and skin-soothing effects.

It's important to exercise caution when using herbal and natural remedies, as their safety and efficacy can vary widely. Before trying any of these treatments, consult with a healthcare professional, particularly one who is knowledgeable about herbal medicine. Also, be mindful of potential allergic reactions or interactions with other medications.

4.4 Mind-Body Practices

Mind-body practices aim to promote overall well-being and manage stress, which can be particularly beneficial for individuals with Morgellons who often experience psychological distress. These practices include:

- **Meditation:** Meditation techniques can help reduce stress, improve relaxation, and enhance mental clarity. Mindfulness meditation, in particular, can be effective for managing anxiety and depression.

- **Yoga:** Yoga combines physical postures, breathing exercises, and meditation to promote both physical and mental well-being. It can enhance flexibility, reduce tension, and improve stress management.

- **Tai Chi:** Tai Chi is a low-impact martial art that emphasizes slow, flowing movements. It can improve balance, reduce stress, and enhance overall physical and mental health.

- **Deep Breathing Exercises:** Deep breathing exercises, such as diaphragmatic breathing or the 4-7-8 technique, can help individuals with Morgellons manage stress and anxiety by promoting relaxation.

- **Biofeedback:** Biofeedback is a therapeutic technique that provides individuals with real-time information about physiological processes like heart rate and muscle tension. It can help individuals learn to control physical responses to stress.

These mind-body practices can be integrated into a comprehensive Morgellons management plan to address the emotional and psychological aspects of the condition. While they may not directly treat the physical symptoms of Morgellons, they can help individuals cope with the stress and anxiety often associated with the condition, ultimately improving their overall quality of life.

CHAPTER 5

Lifestyle Changes

5.1 Personal Hygiene

Lifestyle changes, including adjustments to personal hygiene practices, can be an important aspect of managing Morgellons. While there is no definitive cure for the condition, maintaining good personal hygiene can help reduce the risk of skin complications and provide some relief from symptoms. Here are some recommendations for personal hygiene when living with Morgellons:

- **Gentle Cleansing:** Use mild, fragrance-free soaps and cleansers to wash your skin. Avoid harsh or abrasive products that can further irritate the skin.

- **Warm Water:** When bathing or showering, use lukewarm water instead of hot water, which can worsen itching and dryness.

- **Regular Showering:** Bathing or showering regularly can help keep the skin clean and reduce the risk of skin infections. Pat your skin dry gently with a soft towel after bathing.

- **Nail Care:** Keep your fingernails short and clean to reduce the risk of scratching and creating open sores. Avoid excessive scratching, as it can lead to skin complications.

- **Bedding and Clothing:** Wash your bedding, pillowcases, and

clothing regularly in hot water
to minimize potential irritants.
Use hypoallergenic detergents
and avoid fabric softeners or
fragranced products.

- **Avoid Irritants:** Be mindful of
  any personal care products,
  such as lotions, creams, or
  perfumes, that may irritate your
  skin. opt for hypoallergenic and
  fragrance-free options.

- **Change Clothing:** Change
  your clothing regularly,
  particularly if you experience
  excessive sweating or if your
  clothing becomes soiled or
  contaminated.

- **Environmental
  Considerations:** Ensure that
  your living environment is
  clean and free from potential

irritants or allergens. Regularly clean your living space to reduce dust and other potential triggers.

It's essential to approach personal hygiene practices with care and sensitivity, as individuals with Morgellons often have heightened skin sensitivity. Consulting with a healthcare provider who is knowledgeable about Morgellons can help you develop a hygiene routine that is tailored to your specific needs and symptoms. Personal hygiene, when combined with other treatment strategies, can contribute to better skin health and overall well-being.

5.2 Environmental Considerations

In the management of Morgellons, paying attention to environmental factors is crucial, as certain triggers or irritants in the environment may exacerbate symptoms or contribute to the condition's progression. Here are some important environmental considerations for individuals with Morgellons:

- **Reduce Potential Allergens:** Identify and minimize potential allergens in your living space, such as pet dander, pollen, mold, or dust mites. Regular cleaning and maintaining good indoor air quality can help.

- **Air Filtration:** Consider using air purifiers with HEPA filters to improve air quality in your home, especially in your bedroom. This can reduce exposure to airborne irritants.

- **Clean Living Environment:** Regularly clean and vacuum your home to reduce dust and potential irritants. Use a vacuum cleaner with a HEPA filter to trap smaller particles.

- **Pest Control:** Keep your living space free from pests, as insect bites or infestations can exacerbate symptoms. Consider professional pest control if necessary.

- **Environmental Triggers:** Identify and avoid environmental factors that may worsen your symptoms. For some individuals, exposure to certain chemicals, fabrics, or materials can lead to skin irritation. Being mindful of these triggers is important.

- **Personal Space:** Create a personal space that is comfortable and free from potential irritants. Consider using hypoallergenic bedding and furniture to reduce the risk of skin irritation.

- **Avoiding Contaminants:** Be cautious with potential contaminants in your environment, such as pesticides, harsh cleaning chemicals, or toxic substances. Minimize exposure to these chemicals, and use natural or less irritating alternatives if possible.

- **Temperature and Humidity:**
  Maintain a comfortable indoor
  temperature and humidity level,
  as extreme heat, cold, or low
  humidity can impact skin
  health. Use a humidifier or
  dehumidifier as needed.

- **Outdoor Considerations:**
  When spending time outdoors,
  be mindful of environmental
  factors like sun exposure, heat,
  and allergens. Protect your skin
  from excessive sun exposure
  and stay hydrated in hot
  weather.

It's important to remember that
environmental considerations may
vary from person to person, and not
all individuals with Morgellons will
have the same triggers or sensitivities.
Identifying and managing
environmental factors that exacerbate

symptoms is a personal and ongoing process. Consulting with a healthcare provider or an environmental specialist can provide guidance and support in creating a safe and comfortable living environment for individuals with Morgellons.

5.3 Managing Stress and Anxiety

Stress and anxiety management are essential components of coping with Morgellons, as the condition can be emotionally and psychologically distressing. Strategies to manage stress and anxiety can significantly improve the overall well-being of individuals with Morgellons. Here are some approaches for effectively managing stress and anxiety:

- **Counseling and Therapy:**
Seek support from a mental
health professional, such as a
psychologist or therapist, who
can provide strategies for
managing anxiety, stress, and
emotional challenges.
Cognitive-behavioral therapy
(CBT) and other evidence-
based therapies can be
particularly helpful.

- **Mindfulness and Meditation:**
Practice mindfulness
techniques and meditation to
increase awareness, reduce
stress, and promote relaxation.
Mindfulness can help
individuals learn to cope with
the distressing aspects of
Morgellons more effectively.

- **Relaxation Exercises:** Engage
in relaxation exercises, such as

deep breathing, progressive muscle relaxation, or guided imagery. These techniques can help reduce tension and promote emotional well-being.

- **Physical Activity:** Regular physical activity can be a powerful stress reliever. Exercise releases endorphins, which are natural mood boosters. Consult with a healthcare provider to determine suitable exercise options based on your physical capabilities.

- **Social Support:** Connect with friends, family, and support groups. Sharing your experiences with others who understand the challenges of living with Morgellons can provide emotional support and a sense of community.

- **Time Management:** Develop effective time management strategies to reduce stress related to daily responsibilities and commitments. Setting realistic goals and prioritizing tasks can be beneficial.

- **Hobbies and Distractions:** Engage in enjoyable activities and hobbies that can serve as healthy distractions from Morgellons-related stressors. Pursuing interests and hobbies can improve your overall quality of life.

- **Seek Professional Help:** If stress and anxiety become overwhelming, consider consulting a healthcare provider about medication or other medical interventions to manage these symptoms. In some cases, medication may be necessary to help control anxiety or depression.

- **Educate Yourself:** Gaining a better understanding of Morgellons and its management can reduce uncertainty and anxiety. Knowledge empowers individuals to take control of their health and advocate for themselves within the healthcare system.

Managing stress and anxiety is an ongoing process, and what works best for one person may not be the same for another. It's important to find a combination of strategies that work for you and seek professional guidance when needed. Prioritizing emotional well-being and coping effectively with stress can significantly improve your overall quality of life when living with Morgellons.

CHAPTER 6

Preventive Measures

6.1 Avoiding Triggers

Preventive measures are a crucial aspect of managing Morgellons, as avoiding potential triggers can help reduce the frequency and severity of symptoms. While Morgellons triggers can vary from person to person, here are some general guidelines to consider when trying to minimize exposure to potential exacerbating factors:

1. **Environmental Allergens:** Identify and reduce exposure to common environmental allergens, such as pollen, dust mites, and pet dander, which

can exacerbate skin irritation or allergies. Using air purifiers and allergen-proof bedding may help.

2. **Irritants in Personal Care Products:** Be mindful of personal care products, such as soaps, shampoos, and lotions. Opt for hypoallergenic and fragrance-free options to minimize potential skin irritants.

3. **Fabrics and Clothing:** Select clothing made from natural, breathable materials like cotton and avoid fabrics that may cause skin irritation, such as wool or synthetic materials. Wash clothing with hypoallergenic detergents.

4. **Insect Avoidance:** Take measures to avoid insect bites and stings, as these can trigger or worsen skin symptoms. Use insect repellent and protective clothing when spending time outdoors.

5. **Extreme Temperatures:** Be cautious in extreme temperatures. Hot weather, sun exposure, or cold weather can exacerbate symptoms. Protect your skin from excessive sun exposure and dress appropriately for the weather.

6. **Chemical Exposures:** Minimize exposure to potential skin irritants and allergens, including harsh cleaning products, pesticides, and other chemicals. Use natural or less

irritating alternatives for cleaning.

7. **Psychological Stressors:** Identify sources of psychological stress and work on stress management techniques. Reducing emotional stress can help prevent symptom exacerbation.

8. **Skin Protection:** Use protective clothing, such as long sleeves and gloves, to prevent skin contact with potential irritants. This is especially important if you're working with materials or substances that could trigger symptoms.

9. **Allergen Management:** If you have known allergies, manage them effectively through

avoidance and, when necessary, the use of allergy medications prescribed by a healthcare provider.

10. **Dietary Triggers:** If certain foods or food additives appear to exacerbate your symptoms, consider avoiding them. Maintain a food diary to help identify trigger foods.

It's important to remember that identifying and avoiding triggers can be a personal and ongoing process, as what affects one individual may not affect another in the same way. Keeping a detailed journal of your symptoms and potential triggers can help you and your healthcare provider pinpoint specific factors that may worsen your condition. Additionally, working closely with a healthcare provider who is knowledgeable about

Morgellons can be invaluable in developing a personalized plan for trigger avoidance.

6.2 Protective Clothing and Gear

Protective clothing and gear are essential for individuals living with Morgellons, as they can help prevent skin irritation and minimize exposure to potential irritants or allergens. Here are some recommendations for protective clothing and gear:

1. **Long-Sleeved Clothing:** Wear long-sleeved shirts, blouses, or dresses to cover your arms and minimize skin exposure to potential irritants. Choose lightweight, breathable fabrics

like cotton to reduce overheating.

2. **Long Pants or Skirts:** Opt for long pants or skirts to protect your legs from potential skin irritants. Loose-fitting clothing can also be more comfortable and reduce friction against the skin.

3. **Gloves:** Use gloves when handling materials or substances that could trigger or worsen your symptoms. Nitrile or latex gloves are suitable for various tasks and can prevent direct skin contact with potential irritants.

4. **Protective Footwear:** Wear closed-toe shoes and socks to protect your feet from potential irritants and insect bites.

Choose breathable materials for shoes to prevent overheating.

5. **Hats and Head Coverings:** If your face and scalp are sensitive, consider wearing a hat or head covering to shield your head from sun exposure, insect bites, or other potential triggers.

6. **Sun Protection:** Use sunscreen with a high SPF rating and broad-spectrum protection to shield your skin from harmful UV rays. UV exposure can exacerbate skin symptoms.

7. **Eye Protection:** Wear sunglasses with UV protection to protect your eyes from sunlight and reduce the risk of eye irritation from allergens or environmental triggers.

8. **Protective Masks:** If airborne irritants or allergens are a concern, wearing a protective mask can help reduce inhalation and skin exposure. Masks with filters designed for allergen protection may be useful.

9. **Barrier Creams:** Consider using barrier creams or ointments on exposed skin areas to create a protective barrier against potential irritants. These products can reduce friction and protect the skin.

10. **Personal Protective Equipment (PPE):** If your work or daily activities involve exposure to hazardous materials, consider using appropriate personal protective

equipment, such as gloves, goggles, and masks, as recommended by safety guidelines.

It's important to choose protective clothing and gear that is comfortable and suited to your specific needs and daily activities. While protective clothing can help reduce skin contact with potential triggers, it's also essential to address other aspects of Morgellons management, such as stress reduction, hygiene, and environmental considerations, for a comprehensive approach to managing the condition. Consulting with a healthcare provider knowledgeable about Morgellons can provide guidance on selecting the most suitable protective measures for your individual situation.

6.3 Educating Others

Educating others about Morgellons is an important aspect of managing the condition, as it can help raise awareness, reduce stigma, and create a supportive network for individuals living with Morgellons. Here are some considerations for educating others about Morgellons:

1. **Family and Friends:** Start by educating your close family members and friends about Morgellons. Share information about the condition, its symptoms, and the challenges you face. Encourage open communication and foster understanding among your support network.

2. **Healthcare Providers:** Many healthcare professionals may

not be familiar with
Morgellons, or they may have
misconceptions about the
condition. Provide them with
accurate and up-to-date
information to improve your
interactions with medical
professionals and facilitate
better care.

3. **Support Groups:** Join or
create support groups for
individuals with Morgellons.
These groups can be a valuable
platform for sharing
experiences, coping strategies,
and resources. They also
provide a sense of community
and understanding.

4. **Online Communities:** Engage
with online communities and
forums dedicated to
Morgellons. These platforms

offer opportunities to connect with others who have the condition, share information, and discuss treatment options.

5. **Advocacy:** Get involved in advocacy efforts to raise awareness about Morgellons. Collaborate with patient advocacy organizations, participate in awareness campaigns, and share your story to help dispel misconceptions and promote understanding.

6. **Educational Materials:** Develop or distribute educational materials about Morgellons for your community or healthcare providers. This may include brochures, pamphlets, or digital

resources that provide accurate information.

7. **Mental Health Professionals:** Consider educating mental health professionals about the psychological challenges faced by individuals with Morgellons. This can help ensure that they are better equipped to provide appropriate support and therapy.

8. **Employers and Colleagues:** If your condition affects your work life, inform your employer and colleagues about Morgellons. Discuss any accommodations or adjustments that may be necessary for your job.

9. **Media Outreach:** Share your story with the media if you are

comfortable doing so. It can help raise awareness on a broader scale and potentially lead to increased research and understanding.

10. **Medical Research and Scientific Communities:** Encourage and support research on Morgellons by collaborating with researchers and institutions. By participating in research studies or clinical trials, you can contribute to a better understanding of the condition.

Educating others about Morgellons is a proactive step toward reducing stigma, improving support systems, and increasing understanding of the condition. When engaging in educational efforts, it's important to provide accurate and evidence-based information to dispel myths and misconceptions. By working together to raise awareness and build a supportive community, individuals with Morgellons can find better ways to cope with the challenges they face.

6.4 Maintaining a Positive Outlook

Maintaining a positive outlook when living with a challenging condition like Morgellons is essential for your overall well-being. While Morgellons can be distressing, there are strategies and practices that can help you stay positive and improve your quality of life:

1. **Stay Informed:** Learn as much as you can about Morgellons, its symptoms, and potential

treatments. Understanding your condition can help reduce uncertainty and empower you to advocate for your health.

2. **Set Realistic Goals:** Focus on setting achievable goals for yourself. These can be related to symptom management, lifestyle changes, or emotional well-being. Achieving even small goals can boost your confidence and positivity.

3. **Mindfulness and Meditation:** Practice mindfulness and meditation to stay present and reduce anxiety. These techniques can help you manage stress and enhance your overall mental well-being.

4. **Coping Strategies:** Develop effective coping strategies for

dealing with the emotional and physical challenges of Morgellons. This may involve seeking support from mental health professionals, support groups, or self-help resources.

5. **Self-Care:** Prioritize self-care to ensure your physical and emotional needs are met. Engage in activities that bring you joy, relaxation, and fulfillment.

6. **Support System:** Build a strong support system of friends and family who can provide emotional support and understanding. Open communication can help maintain a positive outlook.

7. **Advocacy and Awareness:** Consider getting involved in

advocacy and awareness efforts for Morgellons. Advocacy can give you a sense of purpose and create positive change in the Morgellons community.

8. **Celebrate Small Wins:** Celebrate your achievements, no matter how small. Every step forward is a reason to acknowledge your progress and maintain a positive attitude.

9. **Focus on What You Can Control:** Morgellons can be unpredictable, but you can control certain aspects of your life, such as your self-care, lifestyle, and emotional responses.

10. **Professional Help:** Don't hesitate to seek professional help for emotional support.

Therapists or counselors can provide strategies to maintain a positive outlook, even in challenging circumstances.

11. **Community and Support:** Connect with others who have Morgellons through support groups or online communities. Sharing experiences and strategies can create a sense of belonging and positivity.

12. **Mind-Body Practices:** Engage in mind-body practices like yoga, tai chi, or deep breathing exercises. These practices can improve your overall well-being and contribute to a positive mindset.

Maintaining a positive outlook is a personal journey, and it's okay to have moments of frustration or discouragement. What's important is your ability to bounce back, adapt, and focus on your well-being. Stay patient with yourself and practice self-compassion as you navigate life with Morgellons.

6.5 Hope for Morgellons Patients

Morgellons is a mysterious and controversial condition characterized by a range of symptoms, including skin lesions, crawling sensations, and the presence of unusual fibers or filaments emerging from the skin. Although the medical community has not reached a consensus on the exact cause of Morgellons, nor have they universally accepted it as a distinct disease, there is hope for Morgellons patients in several aspects. This hope lies in ongoing research, medical advancements, improved understanding, and a holistic approach to managing the condition.

1. **Research and Awareness**: One source of hope for Morgellons patients is the increasing attention and research dedicated to the condition. While there is no definitive cause or cure yet, ongoing studies are shedding light on the various aspects of Morgellons. The increased awareness has led to the collection of more data and the pursuit of a better understanding, potentially paving the way for more effective treatments in the future.

2. **Medical Advances**:
    Morgellons is still a poorly
    understood condition, and it
    may take time for the medical
    community to identify a
    specific cause and effective
    treatment. However, with
    continuous scientific
    advancements, there is hope
    that new diagnostic tools and
    treatments will be developed.
    These advances could
    significantly improve the
    quality of life for Morgellons
    patients.

3. **Patient Advocacy and
    Support**: Hope can also be
    found in the growing network
    of Morgellons patient advocacy
    groups and support
    communities. These groups
    provide a platform for patients

to share their experiences, discuss potential treatments, and access emotional support. The sense of community and the exchange of information can be empowering and comforting for those struggling with Morgellons.

4. **Holistic Approaches**: Some Morgellons patients have found hope in holistic and alternative approaches to managing their symptoms. These approaches may include dietary changes, detoxification methods, stress management, and lifestyle adjustments. While not scientifically proven as definitive treatments, they can help improve the overall well-being of patients and provide a

sense of control over their condition.

5. **Symptom Management**: Even in the absence of a cure, there is hope in managing the symptoms of Morgellons. Medical professionals can help patients find ways to alleviate discomfort, reduce itching, and manage pain. Topical treatments and prescription medications may provide some relief.

6. **Psychological Support**: Morgellons often presents with neuropsychiatric symptoms, including anxiety and depression. Psychological therapy and counseling can offer hope by addressing these mental health aspects. By managing the psychological

impact of the condition,
patients may experience an
improved quality of life.

7. **Community Engagement and Education**: Hope for Morgellons patients can also be found in raising awareness and educating the public and medical professionals about the condition. This can lead to increased empathy, understanding, and a more supportive environment for patients seeking help.

while Morgellons remains a complex and enigmatic condition, there are reasons for hope. Ongoing research, medical advancements, patient advocacy, holistic approaches, and support networks all contribute to the optimism that the lives of Morgellons patients can improve. Though the road to managing Morgellons may be challenging, it is essential for patients and their loved ones to remain hopeful, resilient, and actively engaged in the pursuit of better treatments and, ultimately, a better understanding of this condition.

www.ingramcontent.com/pod-product-compliance
Lightning Source LLC
Chambersburg PA
CBHW050844260726
48660CB00006B/2427